BODY SCRUBS

30 Popular Organic Body Scrubs Recipes That Will Make Your Skin Beautiful

By CARRIE DRESDEN

Table of Contents

Introduction

We normally go to the closest beauty shop to buy body and skin treatments when in fact, we could always make one at home. There are a lot of benefits why you should consider making your own beauty products at home. One of them is the fact that you will know exactly what is going to be in the product you are going to apply on to your skin – we can make sure that they are 100% organic if ever we want to and we can assure that it is not going to harm our skin because we are aware of what our skin is sensitive of and what to avoid. In addition to this, the amount of money you can save when you avoid the expensive brands is truly significant.

In this book, you will learn 30 simple and effective body scrubs to make your skin a lot healthier, smoother, and softer than ever. The ingredients included in each recipe are popular and could be found just right inside your kitchen or your backyard,

Learn these recipes now – I can guarantee you'll be happy with the results you will get in a matter of few weeks or less! These organic body scrubs not just beautify your skin; they also do deep cleansing by stimulating cell renewal and get rid of the dead cells from the surface of the skin. You will get a result that is spotlessly clean and fantastically smooth skin that you just can't get enough of!

Chapter 1: The Basics of Making Your Own Organic Body Scrubs

Most people rely on chemical on a bottle in order to attain the beauty they want to achieve – a bottle of shampoo and conditioner that make your hair shinier and give it more volume, a bottle of lotion that promises to take away your wrinkles, and a bottle of body scrub that convince you it will make your skin look radiant and smoother. But while all these products promise to make you look more beautiful, they normally contain destructive chemicals, unnatural preservatives, and toxins that aren't just only bad for your body but as well as for the environment. Ultimately, these artificial chemicals do more damage than good to you and to nature.

Luckily, there is a simple solution for this – making your own organic beauty products at home with natural ingredients that could easily be found in your kitchen and garden. You really don't need to have any special equipment or talent in order to do this. When making these simple skin beauty products at home, you're not only saving money; it also makes you aware of what products are touching your skin. Please keep in mind that that more than half of all the ingredients that you apply on your skin get into your bloodstream. So, exposing your skin to toxic chemicals for a long time can really do lasting damage to your body. Moreover, these organic solutions offer a better alternative to expensive cosmetic products that normally don't reach your expectations.

You have to remember that the three essential elements of all body scrubs are: (1) exfoliation medium with variable grain size; (2) base oils to sooth and moisturize the skin, and; (3) essential oils for scent therapeutic benefits.

When making your own body scrubs, you can choose the best natural ingredients suitable for you. With the use of some practice, you can make almost any body scrub that you want. On top of saving money, homemade body scrubs could be great gifts – put them in pretty jars, attach labels and ribbons, and send them to your friends and family.

Producing your own skin care product at home like body scrubs is a lot easier than you might be thinking. In this book, you will be given 100% natural body scrub recipes that only take about few minutes to prepare but could make your skin healthy, glowing, and radiant.

Chapter 2: The Use and Benefits of Organic Body Scrubs

The skin requires exfoliation from time to time to be rejuvenated and moisturized. So, scrubbing it's an important part of your everyday routine in terms of body cleansing. Exfoliation can be helpful by revealing the smoother and the supple skin layers after the dead cells get removed. It's important both for men and women. There are a lot of different body scrubs for you to choose from to get rid of the dead cells from your body.

Organic body scrubs normally have the following:

- Exfoliant: It's a rough material that can you get rid of the dead skin cells and uncover the soft and smooth younger looking skin from within. Body scrubs normally have rasping materials such as rice bran, sugar, salt, sugar, jojoba beads, sugar, and ground coffee, among others.

- Oil: It's important in holding the mixture together to help you to apply it to your skin. Some body scrubs have more expensive oils.

- Fragrance: Normally, the scent in the scrubs comes from the high-grade essential oils such as spearmint and rosemary.

Among the different benefits of body scrubs, the most important one is that you are able to get a total spa-like experience at the comfort of your own home. The mixtures within the scrubs exfoliate and soften the skin at the same time. But if you have a sensitive skin you have to be careful with the product usage. There are two ways of using the body scrub. You might like to use it dry before getting into the shower or you might simply get into the shower and then use the body scrub the way you want to. Scrubbing your neck and face can be a really subtle job. These are the sensitive parts of the body and you have to know that these parts are quite vulnerable. You might want to leave the neck and the face part out when you are scrubbing.

Body scrubs that have moisturizing elements can help improve the skin's suppleness and also top-up the natural oils lost by the body from showering frequently. Scrubs can also help to fight stretch marks if they contain good hydration. On top of this, firm exfoliation in rounded movements in the parts that have cellulite can help in supplementing the skin's elasticity, giving you a healthier, smoother skin.

Chapter 3: 30 Recipes That Will Make Your Skin More Beautiful Than Ever

Keeping a good skin may take a lot of hard work. Whenever you get to the shower, you may find the bathroom cabinet full of beauty products. From soothing shaving creams and moisturizing shampoos to fruity face washes and body butter, anyone's cabinet may have it. With all these clutter, do you actually need to have any more addition to all the beauty products you already gave? If you don't have a nice body scrub then the answer is definitely a YES. With all the benefits mentioned above, a body scrub is certainly a must have for anyone who wants to have a beautiful, glowing skin. You don't necessarily need to spend a lot of money on body scrub; with the use of simple ingredients found right within your kitchen, you can make your own personalized body scrub. Below are 30 most popular body scrubs you can easily make at home.

1. Simply SweetOil Body Scrub

Ingredients:
- ½ cup of grounded oatmeal
- ½ cup of brown sugar
- ¼ cup of olive oil
- a few drops of essential oils like lavender or almond oil

Directions:

Mix all the ingredients together to combine thoroughly. It is important not to blend the ingredients into a smooth looking texture; the concoction has to be a bit bristly in order to work fine as a scrub. Put it in a sealed container and keep it in a dry place for at least 3 weeks. Use a quarter-sized amount of scrub on a weekly basis. It will remove the dead skin as well as also lessen blemishes on your skin.

2. Thrilla Vanilla Body Scrub

Ingredients:
- 1 cup brown sugar
- ½ cup almond oil
- ½ tablespoon nourishing vitamin E oil
- 1 tablespoon vanilla extract

Directions:

Combine all the ingredients together, whip them thoroughly and it is ready. This mixture is not only going to make you smell delectably sweet the whole day, but your skin is going to make you feel baby soft as well.

3. Simply Banana Body Scrub

Ingredients:

- 3 tablespoons of granulated sugar
- 1 ripe banana
- ¼ tablespoon of essential oil

Directions:

Combine all the ingredients together. Make sure not to smash the banana all the way because it has to be bristly and not soppy. Apply the mixture copiously throughout your skin. Leave it for about 20 minutes. When your skin begins to stretch, then you can start scrubbing it. The banana scrub is going to work the dirt out without drying up your skin and causing sore of any kind.

4. Rough Coconut Body Scrub

Ingredients:

- 20 drops of lavender oil
- 2 cups of coconut oil
- 1 cup Epsom salt

Directions:

Combine all the ingredients together until they are incorporated well. Keep the mixture in a sealed container until it's ready for use. This organic body scrub is unique compared to others; you'll get the calming effect of lavender oil, the nourishing effect of coconut oil, and magnesium enhancement of Epsom salt, all combined into one.

5. Minty Cocoa Scrub for the Lips

Ingredients:
- ¼ tablespoon cocoa powder
- 1 tablespoon jojoba oil
- 1 tablespoon ultra-fine sugar
- 1 to 2 drops of mint oil

Directions:
Combine the ingredients all together, whip them thoroughly and keep it in an airtight container. Use it on a regular basis for beautiful smooth lips.

6. Fresh Coffee Scrub

Ingredients:
- 1/3 cup of fresh coffee grounds
- ½ cup of sugar
- 1 cup coconut oil
- 2 to 3 tablespoon of olive oil
- 4 to 5 ounces of jelly jars

Directions:

In a bowl, mix the sugar, coconut oil, olive oil, coffee grounds, and make sure that they are incorporated thoroughly. Add the scrub mixture to the jelly jars.

7. Minty Green Tea Body Scrub

Ingredients:

- o 1 tea bag of green tea or approximately a tablespoon of loose green tea leaf
- o 3 tablespoons of baking soda
- o 3 cups of Epsom salts
- o 4 tablespoons of oil of your choice
- o 8 drops of orange essential oil
- o 8 drops of lime essential oil
- o zest from a lemon, lime, or orange

Directions:

Combine the baking soda and Epsom salts together in a large-sized bowl. Add the oil and combine them well. Cut the green tea bag open and pour it into the mixture. Add in the essential oil as well as the citrus zest. Combine everything together and it has to be the constancy of damp packing snow. Scoop out of the bowl and put it into a container and then cover the container. This mixture is a good scrub for the body to keep its natural moisture.

8. Lemon Poppy Seed Body Scrub

Ingredients:

- ¼ cup of cornmeal
- ½ cup of coconut oil
- ½ cup of coconut oil
- 1 tablespoon of poppy seeds
- 1 cup of sugar
- 1 teaspoon of vanilla extract
- ½ cup of coconut oil

Directions:

Zest the lemons, and then allow it to sit in order to dry for about one to two hours. If there is no zester in your kitchen, you can simply remove the lemon peel using a vegetable peeler and then shred the peel using a knife. In a medium sized bowl, combine the sugar, poppy seeds, vanilla, cornmeal, and lemon zest, mix well. Add the oil to the ingredients and continue mixing. Keep the mixture in a sealed jar for up to 3 months before using.

9. Almond Joy Body Scrub

Ingredients:

- ½ cup of coconut oil
- ½ cup of sugar
- ½ cup of almond meal
- 1 tablespoon of unsweetened coconut flakes
- 1 tablespoon of cocoa powder

Directions:

Make sure to use the pre-ground almond meal or grind the almonds using a food processor or high powered blender. If you don't have any of those, you can place the nuts inside a sandwich bag and carefully hit the nuts using a hammer to crush. In a medium size bowl, mix all the dry ingredients. Add the oil to the ingredients and combine thoroughly. Keep in an airtight jar for. This mixture is good for three months.

10. Chai Masala Body Scrub

Ingredients:

- ¼ cup of black tea
- ¼ teaspoon of black ground pepper
- ½ teaspoon of ground cloves
- ½ cup of coconut oil
- ½ teaspoon of ground cardamom
- ½ teaspoon of ground nutmeg
- 1 tablespoon of ground dry ginger
- 1 tablespoon of ground cinnamon
- 1 teaspoon of vanilla extract
- 1 cup of sugar

Directions:

Crush the black tea leaves to pulverize it. If mortar and pestle or coffee grinder is not available in your kitchen, then you can place the tea leaves inside a sandwich bag and hit it using a hammer or roll over using a rolling pin in order to grind the leaves. The spices are available in the market already ground, or you are able to grate them with the use of grater. In a medium size bowl, mix all dry ingredients and together with the vanilla extract well. Add the oil to the ingredients and combine thoroughly. Keep it in an airtight container up to three months. This is a good body scrub for drying up the skin.

11. Java Mint Scrub

Ingredients:
- ½ cup of sugar
- ½ cup of coffee grounds
- ½ cup of coconut oil
- 2 tablespoons of peppermint tea bags or mint leaves

Directions:

If you choose to use fresh mint, remove the leaves from the stalks and lay them on a cookie sheet. Bake them at the lowest temperature for about 1 hour. Allow the leaves to cool down before crumbling them using your fingers to pulverize. If you choose to use peppermint tea bags, on the other hand, you can cut open the bags to use the leaves inside. In a medium size bowl, mix the mint, coffee, and sugar together. Add the oil to the ingredients and combine them thoroughly. Using this organic body scrub, you can easily get rid of the dead skin cell of your body.

12. Deluxe Massage Bar Recipe

Ingredients:
- ½ - 1 ounce of ground adzuki beans
- ½ - 1 ounce of ground almonds
- ½ - 1 ounce of ground rice

- 2 ounces of cocoa butter
- 3 ounces of Shea butter
- 10 to 20 drops of essential oils of your choice

Directions:

Combine the cocoa butter and Shea butter together over low heat or in the microwave or on the stove until they completely become blended. If you have not already ground the beans, almonds, and rice you have to do it first. You have to keep in mind that when blending, you have to grind the pieces to the size depending on your reference. When you are done grinding them, the next thing to do is to add the exfoliator to the butter mixture and stir in thoroughly.

13. Minty Grapefruit Body Scrub

Ingredients:

- ¼ tablespoon of beet juice of any color of your choice
- ½ cup of white sugar
- ½ cup of coconut oil
- 1 tablespoon of grapefruit juice
- 10 drops of peppermint oil
- 25 drops of grapefruit oil
- zest of 1 grapefruit

Directions:

Put the white sugar and coconut oil in a medium size bowl of a stand mixer that has a paddle attachment for an easier solution. Combine together on low speed, until you produce a thick paste texture. Add in the grapefruit juice, grapefruit zest, grapefruit oil, peppermint oil, and lastly the beet juice, if you want, you can combine these ingredients using the mixer. Mix them on low until they are combined well and then turn up the speed to medium for approximately 20 seconds, or until the mixture becomes well blended and you produce a fluffy texture. Keep in a sealed container and refrigerate overnight before using.

14. Buttery Banana Body Scrub

Ingredients:

- 1/4 cup Shea butter
- 1/4 cup coconut butter
- 1/4 cup coconut oil
- 1/4 apricot kernel oil
- 1 ripe banana
- 1 cup of sugar

Directions:

The first step is to combine the Shea butter, coconut butter, apricot kernel oil, coconut oil, and banana together in a blender. Blend all them until you get a very smooth texture. Add a cup of sugar. This mixture is perfect in making your skin look a lot smoother.

15. Simple Oatmeal Body Scrub

Ingredients:

- 1 C. coconut oil
- ½ C. brown sugar
- ½ C. finely ground oatmeal
- 1-2 Tbs. olive oil
- 4-5 4 oz. Jelly jars

Directions:

Using a food processor or a high-powered blender, pulse the oats until they're consistently pulverized. You'll still have some little pieces combined throughout. In a medium size bowl mix the brown sugar, coconut oil, coconut oil, ground oats, and coconut oil together and mix thoroughly. Put the mixture in an airtight container. This mixture can last for about 6 months if kept in a sealed container.

16. Gingerbread Body Scrub

Ingredients:

- 1 tablespoon of honey
- 1 cup of oil of your choice (coconut oil, olive oil, or sweet almond oil)
- 2 tablespoons of mixed spice
- 2 tablespoons of ground ginger
- 2 cups of brown sugar

Directions:

In a medium size bowl, combine all the ingredients together. If you end up with a mixture that is too oily, you can add some more sugar, but if it is too dry, try to add more oil. The amount of spice you are going to add depends on your own reference. There are oils that can mask the scent of the cinnamon and ginger, so simply add more if necessary. This body scrub is perfect if you are having an issue with dry skin.

17. Pink Salt Body Scrub

Ingredients:

- 1 ounce of sweet almond oil
- 2 ounces of coconut oil
- 5 drops of ylang ylang essential oil
- 5 drops of citrus essential oil

- 8 ounces of pink Himalayan sea salt
- 10 drops of rose geranium essential oil

Directions:

In a medium size container, put all the ingredients and combine. If you noticed that the coconut oil needs to be softening, then you might want to warm it up. This mixture is good in making your skin more moisturized and softer.

18. Floral Almond Body Scrub

Ingredients:

- ¼ cup of lavender buds
- ½ cup of a sweet almond oil
- 1 cup of sea salt
- 6 drops of floral oil
- Some fresh flower petals

Directions:

In a medium size bowl, combine all the ingredients. Mix well to make sure that all the essence of every ingredient is incorporated. This body scrub is the perfect solution for exfoliating your skin.

19. Rose Body Scrub

Ingredients:
- 1 teaspoon of coarse sea salt
- 1 tablespoon of jojoba oil
- 1 tablespoons of rose essential oil
- 2 tablespoons of fine sea salt

Directions:

Combine the coarse sea salt and the fine salt together and then add the jojoba oil or any unscented oil of your choice, and then add the rose oil to the mixture to add flowery aroma to the body scrub. The perfect consistency you want is in the middle of wet and dry – not very crumbly, not very oily.

20. Piña Colada Body Scrub

Ingredients:
- 1 cup of dried coconut
- 1 finely grated lemon zest
- 1 cup of Epsom salts
- 2 tablespoons of coconut oil
- 4 drops of vitamin E oil

Directions:

In a medium size bowl, mix all dry ingredients. Then add the coconut oil to wetness level you want and continue mixing. Transfer the mixture to a clean container. Use this organic body scrub on dry skin to exfoliate while you are in the shower.

21. Ginger Detox Body Scrub

Ingredients:

- ½ cup of Epsom salt
- 1 tablespoon of fresh lemon juice
- 1 tablespoon of ginger

Directions:

Combine roughly chopped ginger and ½ cup Epsom salt in a food processor. Pulse a few times until the ginger is ground and combined. Remove to a small bowl and add lemon juice. Put down a towel and apply scrub before your detox bath.

22. Coffee Body Scrub

Ingredients:

- ½ tablespoon of cinnamon
- ½ cup of coconut oil
- 1 cup of ground organic coffee

- 1 tablespoon of vanilla
- 1 cup of organic salt or sugar

Directions:

Melt the coconut oil and let it cool down, but make sure that it is not going to be solidified. Combine all the ingredients together and keep in a sealed jar or container. This mixture is ideal to use on a weekly basis.

23. Vanilla Coconut Body Scrub

Ingredients:

- ½ cup of solid coconut oil
- 1 cup of white sugar
- 1 teaspoon of seeds from vanilla bean pods

Directions:

Using the whisk attachment on your mixer, whip the solid coconut until it gets all soften. Scrape down the sides of the bowl every 5 minutes. Add a cup white sugar and the seeds from the vanilla pod. Whisk the mixture for another minute or two. Keep the mixture in a container and it is ready for use.

24. Blueberry and Coconut Body Scrub

Ingredients:

- ½ cup of organic coconut oil
- 1 tablespoon of frozen dried blueberries
- 1 cup of white sugar
- 1 teaspoon of lemon essential oil

Directions:

To start off, break down the frozen dried blueberries in a medium size bowl. You can use a food processor, a blender, or even your own hands in order to do this. After doing that, add the coconut oil, sugar, essential oil, and option food coloring to the smashed blueberries. Continue mixing until the ingredients are thoroughly combined and the color of the blueberries comes out.

25. Candy Cane Body Scrub

Ingredients:

- ¼ cup of crushed candy canes
- 1 cup of olive oil
- 4 cups of fine white sugar
- 5 tablespoons of peppermint essential oil

Directions:

In a mixing bowl, add the sugar, stir it thoroughly in order to make sure that there are no clumps. The sugar gently exfoliates the skin which makes it softer and smoother. Next thing to do is to add the olive oil to the sugar and continue stirring. The mixture has to look like wet sand that is not very saturated. Olive oil gives the most amazing results while the almond and sunflower oil, on the other hand, are nice options as well. If a cup of oil does not seem to be enough for you, then try adding a quarter cup more.

26. Coffee Cinnamon Body Scrub

Ingredients:
- ¼ cup of sugar
- ¼ cup of coconut oil
- ¼ cup of coffee grounds
- 1 tablespoon of ground cinnamon

Directions:
In a medium size mixing bowl, combine the cinnamon, coffee, coconut oil, and mix them thoroughly to get the desired effect.

27. Fantasy Citrus Body Scrub

Ingredients:

- 1 cup of sea salt
- ½ cup of coconut oil
- ½ cup of brown sugar
- 5 drops of lemon essential oil
- 10 drops of orange essential oil
- 10 drops of grapefruit essential oil

Directions:

Mix the sugar and sea salt together in a jar or any container with a lid. In a heating pan, pour in the coconut oil and wait for the texture to become liquids. As the last step, combine the essential oil and coconut oil mixture on the sugar and sea salt mixture. This body scrub mixture is perfect for those who have rough hands and feet.

28. Cranberry Sugar Body Scrub

Ingredients:

- ¼ cup of sugar
- ¼ cup of sweet almond oil
- ½ cup of frozen cranberries
- 1 teaspoon of vegetable glycerin
- 2 tablespoons of oat powder

- 2 drops of orange essential oil

Directions:

Using a high-powered blender or a food processor, mix the vegetable glycerin, cranberries, and almond oil; but make sure that you pulse them just enough and not turn the cranberries into the pulpy texture. The mixture has to be thick. Pour in the mixture into a medium size bowl and add in the essential oil followed by the sugar. Add some oat powder in order to make a thick mixture perfect for applying on the skin.

29. Easy Cane Sugar Body Scrub

Ingredients:

- ½ cup of melted coconut oil
- 1 tablespoon of vanilla extract
- 1 cup of kosher salt
- 1 tablespoon of vitamin E oil
- 1 tablespoon of almond extract
- 2 cups of cane sugar

Directions:

In a large size bowl, combine all the ingredients together one by one. If necessary, add more liquid or dry ingredients in order to get the consistency you want. The vanilla extract, coconut oil, and the almond extract will all give this sugar scrub a sweet aroma, but you can freely add your own essential oils depending on your preference. Transfer the mixture into a container and make sure to seal it.

30. Peach Passion Sugar Body Scrub

Ingredients:

- 1 ½ cups of sugar
- ½ cup of coconut oil
- 4 to 5 pieces of passion tea bags
- 10 drops of essential oils

Directions:

Cut the peach tea bags open, empty it, and set aside. In a medium size bowl, put the sugar, loose leaf tea leaves, and combine the ingredients together until they are thoroughly mixed. Add coconut oil slowly and stir until the oil covers the mixture completely. Put the mixture inside a sealed container.

Chapter 4: How to Apply Body Scrubs

Using a body scrub is far from being difficult; however, you'll find a lot of things you have to know before using such amazing skin products. The best way of using a body scrub could be to initially apply the body scrub mixture on a sponge or scrubbing cloth.

Using the body scrub is normally done before you get into the shower. When you take a shower or bath, just begin scrubbing the body scrub mixture all over your body. A neck or face scrubs are naturally soothing and you have to read the product label before using it. Since you are using a homemade mixture, it is most suggested to use gentle exfoliates like grounded nuts, almond or sugar and remember not to use coarse exfoliates like sea salt on your neck or face. Hard abrasives can lead to permanent damage to these parts of the body.

When you are using the scrubbing solution on the skin, it's important to move the sponge or cloth in circular movements directed to the heart. Make use of firm and delicate strokes to guarantee that the whole body is treated and covered evenly. Please remember that using too much pressure could harm the skin and lead to irritation.

Take a seat on the edge of the shower in order to easily clean after the scrub treatment. Because most of the people are going to do a scrub treatment in a bathroom where there is a steam, it's possible that moisture can get into the jar of the product. This could lessen the scrubbing solution's shelf life. Make sure that the jar of the body scrub isn't in the bathroom before taking a shower.

An organic body scrub has to be taken out of the jar using a scoop. If there is no scoop around, don't try to apply the scrub using your bare hands. If you extract the scrub using your fingers, bacteria can be formed within the mixture. This can be risky to the health.

One more related question is how do you often have to exfoliate? A lot of people believe that exfoliating every day can make your skin looking younger and radiant. Contrary to this, you have to use exfoliation very carefully. Using scrubs every day can actually harm your skin. Your exfoliation routine must depend on the type and the condition of your skin; but, it is recommended to use a gentle body scrub once in a week in order to get the best results.

You must always remember that when using an organic body scrub in the shower, the water recess can get slippery because of the oil content. Furthermore, the scrub must never scrape the skin and test on a little portion of skin to see if you will have any allergic reactions.

Conclusion

Body scrubs are a definitely nice treat for your skin because they mildly exfoliate, getting rid of all the dead cells, which leaves your skin healthy and glowing and even moisturized. When you learn how to produce body scrubs ideal for the specific needs of your skin, you truly are giving yourself a much necessary makeover.

Worry about not doing your body scrubs correctly – to be honest, they're so simple to make that even a kid could do them. Body scrubs can be made using different ingredients but normally have an abrasive ingredients or other natural ground product along with another form of liquid. There are people who choose to buy their own liquid bases like lotions or shampoos while others like making their own bases from a blend of essential oils, nourishing oils, soap, or fragrance bases. How simple or luxurious you make a scrub entirely depends on you.

There are some things to consider when you knowing how to make a body scrub. First of all, you have to choose what kind of fragrance you want. Essential oils could be a little expensive but you get more than what you pay for. Since they're 100% natural and have oil extracts from organic herbs and plants, they're really concentrated, so a bit goes a long way. Different essential oils are used for different purposes. For example, lavender is well-known to make you feel relaxed, peppermint or citrus invigorates and gives a good night's sleep and sandalwood or patchouli is known to give you an earthy and sensual experience.

In selecting the type of exfoliant to add to your scrubs, it should depend on your type of skin. Salt is normally most ideal for oily skin since it contains a dehydrating effect but must only be used at least once a week. Sugar is ideal for dry skin since it contains a hydrating effect and could be used on a daily basis. Oatmeal is a nice base if your skin is itching since it has a natural soothing effect also, if you mix it with oil like olive and almond, you will have a body scrub that is going to mollify as it gently exfoliates and moisturizes. Coffee works nicely on the normal skin and is exceptional in terms that it helps in shrinking the varicose veins.